Home Care CEO

A Parent's Guide to Managing In-Home Pediatric Nursing

Charisse N. Montgomery, M.A., M.Ed., GPAC

black&blue PUBLISHING

Toledo, Ohio

HOME CARE CEO: A PARENT'S GUIDE TO IN-HOME
PEDIATRIC NURSING

Published by Black & Blue Publishing, LLC
Toledo, Ohio

To comment on this book via email, send your message to the
author at blackandbluepublishing@outlook.com.

ISBN 978-0-9861761-0-4 (paperback)

ISBN 978-0-9861761-1-1 (e-book)

NOTE TO READERS: The suggestions in this book for are not
meant to substitute for the advice of licensed professionals such as
doctors or nurses. The intent of this book is to facilitate effective
partnerships with such professionals. The publisher and author
expressly disclaim any liability for injuries resulting from use by
readers of the methods contained in this book.

This book is dedicated to
my Little Bug and my Butterfly.

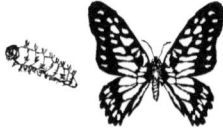

Contents

Acknowledgements

I thank my husband, my son and the rest of my family for the support and motivation to write this book as a resource for families who are starting off with in-home nursing. My husband and my mother were particularly wonderful resources for me during the writing process. My late sister, whose triumphs always seemed to outpace her struggles, is the reason I see the world the way I do and pay special attention to people who are often overlooked. As always, my son Richie is the inspiration for my mission to improve the care of medically fragile children and lighten the loads of their parents. Together, my family composes the symphony that is always playing in my heart.

I am so grateful to the excellent nurses who have worked with Richie over the years. They are essentially the template for the type of excellent care that we have come to expect from all nurses. Kristin Bill, Glenda Mensing, Beth Ringger, Karen Haddad, Libertye Leszkai, Sherice Goodbar, and others have loved our son and managed his needs expertly. They see beyond his medical complexity and appreciate who he is as a person. They will always have a place in our lives because of the way they have cared meticulously for Richie and supported our family. I wish all families with in-home nursing for a medically fragile child could have nurses like these amazing women.

To the members of the many online boards and Facebook groups for parents of children with special needs, I thank you. Many of the conversations I engaged in with these group members showed me the tremendous need for a book like this. I also thank the parents who served as a focus group for making sure this book would meet the needs of other parents who need in-home nursing for their children.

Finally, I am simply thankful. In the great tornado of life, things sometimes seem out of control, and we can't see where we are going. But sometimes, when the storm passes and the dust settles, things have landed into place beautifully. Even though our journey as parents of a medically fragile child began with emotional turmoil, it has since become a purposeful odyssey that brings meaning and depth to our lives. This is the road we were born to travel.

Preface

It is estimated that over 5.9 million children in the U.S. meet the definition of medically fragile. They live with chronic illnesses, including feeding disorders, respiratory illness, seizures or other intellectual or physical disabilities and rely upon technology such as ventilators and feeding tubes[1]. When your child has multiple disabilities and medical complications, your world is complex, to put it mildly. The medication schedules, therapy visits, medical specialists and your child's individual needs are a whirlwind, and you have to manage it all to ensure the best outcomes for your child. With emotions ranging from fear, grief and anger to happiness and relief, the process of bringing home a child who needs in-home care can be complicated. Organizing your child's care is one way to gain some control during a time that can seem confusing and chaotic. Learning to manage your child's care over the long term can relieve a lot of the stress associated with caring for a medically fragile child.

Caregiver Stress

Having a medically fragile child can affect a household greatly, from the financial resources required for therapies and medical treatments to the family structure and economic status. Twenty-two percent of families with medically fragile children have a family member leave the work force in order to care for the child[2]. The divorce rate among parents of medically fragile children is as high as 80%, compared to 50% among parents of typically developing children[3]. The statistics are a little startling, which is a strong argument for considering long-term care. Many medically fragile children qualify for some form of long-term care, and their parents often have the option to select in-home nursing as a way to provide that care. When it is managed effectively, in-home nursing can become a support for caregivers and families stressed with the care of a medically fragile child, while also allowing the child to remain integrated in the community and the parents to continue gainful employment that supports the economic wellbeing of the family.

In-home nursing is different from the care a child receives in a hospital. Parents are required to take on a new role when it comes to in-home nursing, the role of a CEO guiding the team toward a mission of excellent care. This book will benefit parents and caregivers who are new to in-home nursing as well as those who want to increase the efficiency of their nurses or hone their ability to manage the staff of nurses in their homes.

The Author's Personal Experience

I wrote this book because it is exactly what I needed as my family embarked on the home nursing journey. My son was born with a muscle condition called a myopathy, and this genetic condition has a host of effects on his body. It affects his ability to swallow, so he has a feeding-tube (g-tube). It affects his ability to breathe, so he has a tracheostomy. It affects his ability to support his body, so he has a TLSO (thoracic lumbar sacral orthotic) and AFOs (ankle foot orthotics). It affects his ability to move on his own, so he has a wheelchair, a stander, and many other orthopedic and therapeutic devices. His needs were such that we could not manage them without in-home nursing. As the time drew near for his discharge from the hospital after his trach and g-tube surgery, we could have used a guide like this one to help us figure out how to navigate this new world.

My sister, who was born with the same condition as my son, also used in-home nursing. Her advice as I started this journey was very insightful, and I watched her and helped her work through issues with nursing into her adulthood. She passed away in 2012 at the age of 27, and I know that she would be proud of this book and my desire to help parents and families of medically fragile children.

What makes me think I'm qualified to write this book? In our experience of in-home nursing, we have had successes and failures. We have had to let go of dozens of nurses, but we have found some excellent ones who have provided wonderful care for our son for years. I am connected to several online groups for parents of children with disabilities, and in-home nursing is a perpetual topic. Some hate it, some love it and most have horror stories. While we have had some nightmares, we are successful because we are able to approach in-home nursing with a business sense that makes us focus, always, on the mission: excellent care for our son.

I also write from the perspective of my academic credentials. I have a master's degree in Educational Psychology, and my graduate research was focused on ways to provide information to the parents of children with disabilities in order to improve their children's health outcomes. I am a certified Patient Advocate with a strong understanding of the legal aspects of healthcare. I serve on the Family Advisory Council of the local children's hospital where our son receives most of his care, and I mentor other parents who are embarking on this journey. I also serve on our county's Board of Developmental Disabilities. Since our son was born, I have been approached frequently by parents seeking advice about caring for a child with disabilities or significant medical needs. In addition to writing *Home Care CEO: A Parent's Guide to Managing In-Home Pediatric Nursing*, I have written for *Complex Child* e-magazine and *The Mighty*. I also write a blog series called *Teachable Moments* for ProMedica HealthConnect and maintain a personal blog site at madvocator.com.

This book is essentially a compilation of the advice I give to other families who need in-home nursing. I wanted to share this information more broadly because I believe that an informed parent or caregiver becomes empowered, and empowerment can lead to the best care for our children.

How This Book Can Help You

Each chapter in this book focuses on tools and information that will help you to understand your role as a CEO in your home nursing setting. We begin with a quick overview of the history and basics of in-home nursing care and explore the positive and negative aspects. We then explore how to manage in-home nursing from the perspective of a CEO, from finding and selecting nurses to organizing your home in a way that supports the nurses and the care your child receives. Finally, we cover how to handle difficult situations and how to continue the learning process to support your child's health and care. You will also find a few helpful tools in the Resources section at the end of the book: a guide to help you organize a communication book for your home, a quick reference list of interview questions to ask nurses, and a free download of an hour-by-hour schedule chart to display medications and activities.

Throughout this book are personal stories about how our family manages in-home nursing. You will find those stories in italics, in sections that look like this.

As parents, we owe it to our children to give them the best start we can give, so here we are, together, on this journey. It is my sincere hope that you use this book to get excellent care for your child so that he or she may thrive, regardless of diagnosis or ability level. I hope that, like me, you learn to approach this journey with an open mind, an open heart, and a sense of humor. I invite you to correspond with me online through madvocator.com, on social media @madvocator, or via email at madvocator@gmail.com.

I wish you wellness.

Website: www.madvocator.com, www.HomeCareCEObook.com

Email: madvocator@gmail.com

Twitter: www.twitter.com/madvocator   @madvocator

Facebook: www.facebook.com/madvocator

Pinterest: www.pinterest.com/madvocator

Instagram: www.instagram.com/madvocator   @madvocator

CHAPTER 1

Basics of In-Home Nursing

Long-term care is a variety of services that help people with health or personal needs and activities of daily living over a period of time. Long-term care can be provided at home, in the community, or in various types of facilities, including nursing homes and assisted living facilities[5].

Here's a quick rundown of how home nursing works and why it came to exist in the first place. When the Social Security Act was changed in 1965, the importance of providing health care and long-term care to people with disabilities came into focus. This was an attempt to help those who were less able to help themselves.

In-home nursing care is a form of long-term care. Long-term care also includes nursing homes and assisted living facilities. The largest portion of in-home skilled nursing services is paid for through Medicare and Medicaid, federal programs that provide support for the elderly and people with disabilities and/or limited resources. People can also pay for long-term care services out of pocket or through other types of insurance. While Medicaid is funded by the United States government, each state decides how to manage the program under the federal guidelines. Because states manage Medicaid differently, the coverage and qualifications differ based on the state in which you live. Certain parts of Medicaid coverage, listed below, are mandatory no matter where you live[4].

Mandatory Medicaid Services

Inpatient hospital services

Outpatient hospital services

EPSDT: Early and Periodic Screening, Diagnostic, and Treatment Services

Nursing Facility Services

Home health services

Physician services

Rural health clinic services

Federally qualified health center services

Laboratory and X-ray services

Family planning services

Nurse Midwife services

Certified Pediatric and Family Nurse Practitioner services

Freestanding Birth Center services (when recognized by the state)

Transportation to medical care

Tobacco cessation counseling for pregnant women

Waiver

Many states use a waiver program that provides Medicaid coverage to people who traditionally would not be eligible. A waiver could allow Medicaid coverage in certain geographical areas or to children with a particular set of medical needs. Depending on the state, there are other waivers for which only the income of the child is considered as a qualifier for Medicaid benefits, as long as the child meets certain medical qualifications. For specific information regarding your state's program, visit Medicaid.gov and search for Home and Community-Based Waivers.

A number of guidelines are used to determine whether your child is eligible for in-home nursing care through a waiver program. The level of care needed and types of tasks required for that level of care determine your child's eligibility. Most states differentiate between skilled nursing and unskilled nursing care.

When your family is interviewed to determine your eligibility for nursing care through waiver, always describe your child's needs based upon his or her worst day. This means that you describe the worst-case scenario in terms of your child's care and the time and effort it takes to manage this care. After all, you want nurses who can handle the worst day, so you have to describe what that looks like to the people who determine what type of care your child will receive.

Skilled versus non-skilled care

According to the U.S. Department of Health and Human Services, skilled care usually requires the services of a licensed professional such as a nurse, doctor, or therapist[5]. Personal care, on the other hand, is non-skilled care, such as help with bathing, dressing, eating, getting in and out of a bed or chair, moving around, and using the bathroom[5]. The type of care assigned to your child will depend on your child's individual needs, which are based on doctors' orders and family interviews. For example, the care for a child with a trach is typically considered skilled care, and caring for a trach is part of the training for licensed practical nurses and registered nurses.

Positive aspects of in-home nursing care

Let's start with the positive aspects of in-home care. These are simple to define and invaluable for the families who use in-home nursing care for their medically fragile children.

Support and Relief

An exhausted parent can't provide the best care, although occasionally, we have all had to do so. Having an extra set of hands pitch in, especially when you may not have the family support to go it alone, is wonderful. Having someone you trust to help care for your child allows you to rest, work, sleep, run errands and recharge so that you can continue providing excellent care for your child.

> *When our son first came home from the hospital, we lived far from all our family members. Even family and friends who lived within a few hours were not able to assist with our son's care, so we were the only people who could provide care for him. Without family support, we desperately needed the help of in-home nursing and the relief of having someone with more experience dealing with needs like our son's.*
>
> *This was particularly important because we both had successful careers that we wanted to maintain in order to support our family and enrich our lives. Although it is not always perfect, in-home nursing has made that goal possible. Thankfully, our jobs also provide some flexibility, which allows us to manage the days when nurses are sick or unable to work.*

At times, the complicated care required by children with medical needs can be overwhelming. Some children have such complex care that they would need to be institutionalized if not for having in-home nurses. Children who receive in-home nursing often have better health outcomes because of the participation of a medical professional in their daily care.

Love and Connection

Yep, the mushy stuff. Great nurses can become friends and family. They love your child and your family, and you and your child love them back. The more love and support your child receives, the richer his or her life becomes, and nurses can certainly add to the circle of love surrounding your child.

Knowledge and Expertise

Your child's in-home nurses can answer many of your questions about your child's care. Their experience with medically fragile children means they come to your home knowing a lot of things that you will be experiencing for the first time. They can help you to determine if something your child is experiencing is normal or whether it requires a doctor's attention. Nurses are your in-home medical experts. While you should certainly consult a physician for some types of problems, a nurse's clinical knowledge can provide guidance as well.

Even though the positive side of in-home nursing doesn't take up a lot of space on the page, it is priceless to those who experience the love, support and relief provided by great nurses.

Negative aspects of in-home nursing care

Now for the negative aspects of in-home nursing: these are typically the horror stories and complaints you will find among experienced parents. Online groups are filled with accounts of bad nurses and bad situations, some of which cause parents to abandon in-home nursing entirely. We will address how to work through many of these negative aspects in the coming chapters.

Loss of privacy

There's no way around it; having nurses in your home means you have to sacrifice some of your privacy. Gone are the days of munching popcorn on the couch in your undies – at least while the nurse is working. Having nurses in your home is kind of like having company over every day. There are times when this can feel awkward and intrusive, especially early on. After all, it's kind of strange to know that while you sleep, someone is walking around in your home.

Losing some privacy at home is the trade-off for getting your child the care he or she needs and the rest and relief you need. After a while, you get accustomed to having someone else in your home, and when you're exhausted or you've had a rough day, you will want to roll out a red carpet when the nurse arrives.

> *Even though you can't help but lose some part of your family's privacy when nurses are working in your home, you can choose to keep some areas of your home private so that you can retain some of your privacy. In our home, our bedroom is that space. We keep the door closed, and nurses do not enter it. It's our little oasis that belongs to only our family. I encourage you to identify a room in your house that can be an oasis of privacy.*

Inexperienced or incompetent nurses

Inexperienced nurses often give themselves away by freaking out when they should be managing a situation calmly. Just because a nurse has years of experience doesn't mean that nurse has experience with the particular health matters your child is dealing with. Nurses without the proper experience are prone to panicking and making mistakes, as any of us would if we were in over our heads. It's important to realize that many medical errors can occur when the medical professional lacks the experience to do what is required or doesn't know or understand the procedures. Depending on your child's needs, you may require nurses with lots of experience in some aspects of your child's care. Later in this book, we will discuss more about how to select nurses with the appropriate level of experience to handle your child's needs.

Nurses behaving badly

The scariest, ugliest stories about in-home nursing usually are the result of nurses demonstrating a lack of professionalism, bad morals or a disregard for the child for whom they are providing care. Everything from theft, sleeping on the job, frequent tardiness or absence, and basic sloppiness can create in-home nursing nightmares for parents. While these are the stories we hear about the most, they don't represent the hard-working, diligent, caring people who make up the world of in-home nursing. There are definitely bad nurses out there, but many more are good people who want to help your child reach his or her potential and stay well. Unfortunately, the bad apples make it harder for the good nurses.

People have real horror stories with in-home nursing. While some of these awful accounts of in-home nursing are not foreseeable, many more could be prevented. Horror stories often happen when parents are not prepared to manage and direct their child's care like a CEO manages a company. Once you open your home to nursing, you essentially become the employer of a small staff, even if you aren't signing the paychecks. As in any workplace, the staff needs to know the rules and expectations, and it is your job to set them and communicate them well. This is your new job; you've been promoted to Home Care CEO.

CHAPTER 2
Your Role as a Home Care CEO

The CEO of a company is its chief executive officer. CEOs are responsible for leading all aspects of a successful business, including management of the work environment, employees, and working toward the mission of the company. The major tasks you are responsible for as a Home Care CEO are explained below.

Leadership

Leadership is the CEO's main job. No one knows your child better than you do, so you are the primary source of information about your child's health and the primary contact for the various physicians, caregivers and services associated with your child's care. You set the tone for your child's care and the expectations others have for your child.

Setting the mission and guiding everyone to achieve it

Many times, the first role of a CEO is to establish and communicate the company's mission. As a Home Care CEO, you are responsible, first and foremost, for your child's care, which is your "company's" primary mission. All other obligations are secondary to the mission of ensuring the best care possible for your child. Creating a mission statement is simple.

Our mission is to provide excellent care for _____.

The mission of excellent care is your goal, and making sure that everyone is working toward it requires management skills and focus.

Secondary goals

You may also want to set secondary goals for your child that deal with medical or developmental issues. Don't be afraid to declare your goals and even post them so they are visible. I think of the factories that have a sign saying "Accident free for _ _ _ days!" Let everyone involved in your child's care be aware of where you're going next. They can all offer support and assistance in getting there.

- No hospitalizations this year
- Finish potty training by June
- Learn the alphabet in three months
- Get rid of the ventilator by Spring
- Help ___ in his/her goal to become a scientist

Obviously, some of these goals require the support of physicians as well as the nurses in your home. Make sure your child's doctors are aware and on board with your goals.

Each of the following roles of a CEO will be discussed in the chapters that follow, including ways you can apply these skills to become the CEO of your child's care.

Managing the work environment

You are responsible for the needs of your nurses as employees, and making sure their work environment is safe is an important part of managing these needs. You are also responsible for making sure the nurses have the tools they need to perform their jobs effectively.

Getting the right people in place

What good is a CEO without great employees? Finding and keeping great nurses is especially important to the mission of excellent care.

Communicating with your child's nurses

Communication is the skill that will allow you to get everyone else on board with your mission. Not only do you have to communicate with the nurses, you are also responsible to the state or insurance company's policies for in-home nursing and, if you use a nursing agency, you are responsible to uphold the agency's rules and guidelines and communicate with their office employees as needed.

Remaining informed

Most people underestimate how much leadership and learning are connected. Staying up-to-date on treatments, equipment, research and current events can help you to identify ways to provide better care for your child.

Once you know where you are going, you can work on the path to get there. First, you have to create a space for your nurses to work and for your child to be cared for safely.

CHAPTER 3

Managing the work environment

Safety

For your child's nurses, your home is their workplace. As the Home Care CEO, your first job is to make sure their workplace is safe. With the responsibilities we have for our children, it is hard to maintain a spotless home, but safety is very important. The safety of nurses includes everything from removing items that can cause a nurse to trip and fall to managing temperature and pest control.

Childproofing the home in a way that is appropriate for your child is also part of creating a safe environment.

Because our child does not walk or crawl, we didn't need to do traditional childproofing like locking cabinets or oven knobs. However, we do have to remain constantly vigilant about small items that fall on the floor. Making sure our son is safe reduces the opportunities for emergency situations that the nurses or we will have to handle.

Making sure your home is safe also reduces the chance for accidents that could cause injury to the nurses or to your child. Keeping a safe home may also help you to keep great nurses; great nurses want to work in safe places. Nurses who don't care about the safety of your home may also lack concern about their own safety or the safety of your child.

Lighting

Lights are an important aspect of safety. Nurses need to be able to see where they are going and what they are doing, especially when it comes to giving medications and performing medical procedures like injections or tube feedings.

Overnight, lighting is even more important, since low lighting can make it easy for a nurse to fall asleep, but too much light can prevent your child from sleeping well. You will need to decide how much light is appropriate in the room where your child sleeps, and you may have to test different light sources, such as closet lights, hallway lights or lamps.

In our home, a lamp with one 60-watt bulb stays on in our son's room at night. Our son can sleep with that amount of light on, and the nurse can stay awake and see well for the tasks she needs to complete. We also provide a little book light near the bed for additional task lighting when it is needed.

Rules for access

Many big corporate buildings require access cards to get into certain parts of the building. In your home, you will need to determine which parts of the home are open to nurses and which ones are not. The access to different parts of your home depends on your home's size and layout, your feelings about privacy, and the needs of your child. Once you decide where nurses can and cannot go in your home, be sure to communicate this to the nurses on day one.

Our bedroom, for example, is off limits to the nurses in our home. We like keeping this area private, and the door remains closed. Our kitchen is far from our son's room and on a different floor of the house. For that reason, we placed a mini-

fridge and microwave in our son's room for the nurses to use, which allows them to stay close to him. Since it isn't easy to move our son from room to room, the nurses are expected to be close enough to hear him and the alarms on his equipment. If your child moves from room to room a lot, or if your home is compact, your ideas about access may be more liberal.

Security

Managing the security of your home is a matter of safety for your family and your nurses. Do the external doors remain closed and locked? Does the nurse have access to a key when she or he takes your child out of the home? Are you willing to give nurses your alarm code? Does the nurse ring the doorbell to come into the home at the beginning of each shift? These are questions you will need to consider based on the area where you live and your feelings about home security.

Having spent a portion of my adulthood in a city with a high crime rate, my preference is to limit the access of non-family members to keys and alarm codes. We let the nurses in when they arrive for their shifts and lock the door after they enter. We have one house key on a giant key ring that can be used when a nurse needs to leave the home with our son, and we are careful to make sure it is returned each time it is used. We choose not to be too trusting with keys and alarm codes, as they affect our safety and security as a family.

Emergency Plans

Emergency exits and plans should be thought out carefully. If your child has an emergency bag, the nurse should know where to find it and know how to access all exits from the home. While you hope the nurse never has to flee the home due to an emergency, you want to be sure that the nurse is prepared to do so if necessary.

Medication safety

Ensuring that all medications, controlled substances in particular, are in places that cannot be accessed by children is important to consider when organizing your home. If your child takes controlled substances, you will need a procedure for counting and verifying the number of doses left at the end of each shift. This protects your child, the nurses, and other children in your home. Your procedure might even include having a third person present when medications are administered.

Cameras

Having cameras in the home is the single most important piece of advice that I give to families before they begin in-home nursing. Many businesses use cameras to help manage the safety of the workplace and the productivity of the employees. Cameras can be one of the most important tools to keep your child safe.

We chose a two-camera DVR system that we set to record during our scheduled nursing shifts; our system also allows us to log in remotely and view our son's room on a live feed. Every nursing shift is recorded, so all nurses are treated fairly. The cameras are visible, which was really important to us. Our goal is not to catch a nurse after she or he has done something wrong; instead, we want to prevent these things from happening in the first place. For that reason, we inform all nurses about the cameras. I have found that good nurses are not concerned about the presence of cameras.

Unfortunately, we have experienced a situation in which a nurse neglected and abused our son during an overnight shift.

This happened even with her awareness of the cameras. Because of the cameras, we were able to identify the behavior within hours of the nurse's shift, and we were able to take action. Chapter 5 has more information on how to handle these types of situations.

Tips about cameras
- Change the password from the factory setting to prevent public access to your camera feed.
- Get a portable hard drive if you are using a DVR system; the DVR device doesn't have a lot of memory, and you will need extra memory to save the recordings. You may wish to delete the recordings after a certain amount of time.
- Do not place cameras in the bathroom; it's illegal.
- While every state allows the use of cameras or "nanny cams," state laws about audio recording can vary. If your video system includes audio recording, California, Connecticut, Delaware, Florida, Hawaii, Illinois, Louisiana, Maryland, Massachusetts, Montana, Nevada, New Hampshire, Oregon, Pennsylvania and Washington require you to inform your nurses. I highly recommend providing this information in writing and asking nurses to sign a document that says they know about it; this can protect you legally.

Workplace supplies

Every workplace requires supplies, and as a Home Care CEO, it is your job to make sure your nurses have what they need to perform their jobs. Any medications your child takes, along with medical supplies used for your child's care, will need to be available to the nurses at all times. These supplies may come from a durable medical equipment (DME) supplier, the nurse or agency may provide them, or you may need to purchase them.

Making sure that all supplies are ordered regularly and that all medications are stocked can require a bit of organization. To do this efficiently, you can order supplies and prescriptions on the same day of each month. Nurses often help with organizing or putting away durable medical equipment and medical supplies.

Organizing supplies well helps nurses find what they need quickly, which is essential in an emergency situation. Families might use clear plastic bins and drawers, over the door shoe racks, and shelves to store supplies. Labeling the drawers is very helpful, especially for nurses who are new to your home.

Furniture

The nurse will require, at a minimum, a chair to sit in. A table or countertop where medications and food can be prepared is also helpful.

Other supply items

Nurses will need access to trashcans, a refrigerator for medications and food (if needed), gloves, paper towels, hand sanitizer and toilet paper. Depending on the layout of your home, you may wish to have a small refrigerator and microwave in or near your child's room so the nurse will have easy access to them.

Final thoughts on the work environment

Creating an environment that makes the nurse's job easier will help you attract and keep the best nurses, much like great benefits and perks keep employees happy with their jobs at large corporations. Being thoughtful about the comfort and needs of the people who work in your home is a characteristic of a great Home Care CEO.

18

CHAPTER 4

Getting the right people in place

The most important part of your job as a Home Care CEO, and the most important aspect of securing the best care for your child, is selecting the right nurses.

Finding a good nurse is not just about checking off a list of skills the nurse can perform; it's also about finding someone who is a good fit for your home. Having consistent nurses who know your child well contributes to the best care for your child. That's why it is important to identify good nurses who can provide continuity by staying around for the long haul, whenever possible. A revolving door of nurses is not good for you or your child, so finding and keeping good nurses is the goal.

You don't have to be besties with your child's nurse, but sometimes personalities don't mix well, or you just annoy each other. Having a nurse with whom you don't get along doesn't bode well for long-term success. Weeding out nurses who are not a good fit, before you waste time training them and before your child develops attachments to them, is essential to managing your child's medical and emotional needs.

We will focus on licensed practical nurses (LPNs) and registered nurses (RNs), since they provide skilled care, but the information provided can be applied to the selection of any type of home nurse or health aide.

Most people either select nurses from agencies or use private duty independent providers. I have heard parents debate over whether independent nurses or agency nurses are better; we have found great nurses from both sources (and not so great ones from both sources).

Independent Providers

Independent nurses are self-employed nurses who are able to work in the home setting. Lists of nurses who are permitted to provide care as independent nurses are available through waiver case managers, social workers and state-run websites for home care. Because independent nurses work for themselves as independent contractors, they manage their own schedules, and they bill the state or the county for the hours they work. LPNs have to work under the supervision of a registered nurse, and that RN is required to make regular visits to the home to check on the quality of care that is being provided. These visits are required at specific intervals.

The state or county periodically audit nurses to be sure that they are following proper procedures and conducting their visits on time. Take caution if an RN supervisor asks you to backdate any forms and signatures. This is a violation and can put your home nursing status at risk if you are found to have falsified information by backdating a signature. It is the responsibility of the nurses to make sure that their supervisory visits are conducted on time.

Agencies

Nursing agencies are businesses that employ multiple nurses, usually LPNs and certified nursing assistants (CNAs). These nurses, like independent nurses, are supervised by a registered nurse who is required to make regular home visits.

20

Good agencies will send nurses for a meet and greet so you can talk to the nurse and find out about that nurse's experience and qualifications before you make a decision to have him or her work in your home. The better-staffed agencies also allow job shadowing and orientation so the nurse can become familiar with your routine and your child. You should always expect and demand that the agency communicate with you regularly and respond quickly to your concerns.

Setting the schedule

You will need to decide when you want to have nurses in your home. This will be partially determined by the number of hours per week for which your child qualifies for in-home nursing and partially dependent on your family's schedule. Decide when you most need nursing support and how that support will affect your family's schedule.

The interview

The interview offers you a chance to get to know more about nurses and to screen for possible concerns about the quality of their work and their work ethic. A series of common questions is listed below, along with how to interpret the answers. Make note of how each question relates to the mission of providing excellent care for your child.

In general, you will get much more information from open-ended questions than from yes/no questions. For example, instead of asking, "have you ever taken care of a child with a tracheostomy?," which is a question that will generate a yes or no, ask the nurse to tell you about a case that required him or her to care for a child with a tracheostomy. The nurse will provide more

21

information than a yes or no, and you will gain a better understanding of the nurse's level of experience.

Note: Many nurses who work in home care refer to their patients as "cases." That is the term used in the interview questions that follow. It seems a little impersonal, but it's the jargon of the home nursing trade.

Introducing your child

I begin nurse interviews by providing a background on my son's condition, his progress and his needs. This provides some direction for the nurse so she or he will understand what skills I am looking for in a nurse and what experience the nurse might need to be a good fit in our home.

Tell me about yourself.

This question allows nurses to introduce themselves and highlight the aspects of their experience that are relevant. Listen for years of experience, where that experience took place (nursing home, home care, hospital, etc.), the types of equipment they have used and medical care they have provided (tracheostomy, tube feeding, etc.).

Tell me about your experience caring for a child with _____.

Fill in the blank with the equipment, medical devices or specific condition of your child. Many families prefer to work with nurses who have experience with their child's needs and the equipment their child uses; others prefer or don't mind training nurses on their child's care or on the use of certain equipment. You will need to decide what is best for you and your child.

In our home, we prefer seasoned nurses who have seen a lot, but some families find this intimidating or feel that a very experienced nurse will override their decisions. Because we take on the CEO role, we have not had difficulty with nurses offering unsolicited advice or overruling our decisions, but that can happen and it often depends on the personalities involved. We have found that, for our son, inexperienced nurses simply didn't have the expertise to make fast judgments in emergency situations, but that is truly a matter of preference for each family.

Tell me about your pediatric experience.

Not everyone will find it necessary for nurses to have pediatric experience. Depending on your child's age or complexity of your child's medical issues, this question may or may not be relevant to you.

Because our son came home with a trach, vent and other equipment at four months old, it was important for us to know that the nurses we hired were not only comfortable with the trach and vent, but also comfortable with managing them on a tiny baby. Some nurses were visibly very nervous about handling a child of his size, and those nurses were not the best fit for our home.

What do you like most and least about home nursing?

This question just helps you to understand the nurse's personal motivation for working in the home setting. If they like home care just for the money, for example, that might be a red flag.

Why did you leave your last case? Have you ever been fired or asked to leave a case?

Television host Dr. Phil says "the best predictor of future behavior is past behavior." Understanding a nurse's past conflicts or situations that caused the nurse to leave a case may tell you a lot about how that nurse would work in your home.

Thinking about the families you have worked with in the past, what would they say about your attendance and timeliness?

This is another example of how past behavior might indicate future behavior.

Can you tell me about a time when you dealt with an emergency with a patient? What happened, what did you do, and what was the outcome?

Getting an idea of the types of emergency scenarios a nurse has encountered is the purpose of this question.

> *We had a nurse who considered vomiting a serious emergency, and she panicked and screamed whenever our son vomited. Needless to say, she was not ready for prime time.*

Listen for clues about how calm the nurse was during the situation or how she or he thought out a plan for handling the emergency. This will help you to determine whether the nurse will be able to handle the types of emergencies you might anticipate with your child.

What is your availability to work? Are you willing to fill in for other nurses if necessary? Are there days or times when you are absolutely not available?

Part of your job as a Home Care CEO is to make sure that you have all the shifts filled to your satisfaction. Making sure the nurse can work when you need her or him will help you to plan a schedule that works for your needs. A nurse who is not willing to chip in when someone else needs time off might not be the best choice for your home.

Some nurses prefer days shift, while others prefer second or third shift. Knowing which shift a nurse prefers will help you with scheduling and allow you to select people who are at their best during a particular time of day.

> *Once, when we were looking for third shift nurses, we interviewed a nurse who usually worked days but needed work. She said, "I don't like night shift, and I might fall asleep, but I'm a light sleeper." She obviously was not suited for the shift we needed to fill, not to mention that she was unprofessional for predicting that she would be asleep on the job. Next!*

Besides carrying out the doctor's orders in the care plan, how else do you assist or support the children and families on the cases you work?

Good nurses follow the orders on their care plans; great nurses find other ways to support the family. Many nurses who are experienced in pediatric home care understand that it's not just about following a schedule of medical procedures. Great nurses add value to their presence and make your family life easier and better.

> *In our home, the nurses we value the most have gone above and beyond to make our lives easier. Sometimes they fold laundry, wash dishes or do art projects with our son. These*

types of activities, though not required, add value to the nurse's presence in our home and in our lives.

Tell me about a situation where you disagreed with a parent about the appropriate way to care for their child. How did you handle it?

As the Home Care CEO, you have to know whether you have a team player or a ball hog on your hands. Knowing whether the nurse is able to follow your lead and how she or he will act when there is a disagreement is very important. While you may choose to welcome the input of nurses, you are ultimately the one in charge of your child's care.

Beware of nurses who talk negatively about families they have worked with in the past. We interviewed one nurse who talked on and on about what idiots the parents were on her past four cases. Her disrespect for the parents and her willingness to tell us about it showed a lack of professionalism that we didn't want to invite into our home. Badmouthing families is a bad habit, and your family will probably be next if you choose a nurse who does it.

Do you smoke?

Smoking might not be a deal-breaker in every home, but if your child has acute respiratory issues, it's a good idea to find out the smoking status of your nurses. It is well researched and documented that second- and third-hand smoke[7,8] can have a negative impact on health, especially among those with other health issues.

We prefer nurses who do not smoke. In the past, we have hired nurses who smoked, but it seemed that no matter how hard they tried, they or their belongings smelled of smoke, and where there's smoke, there are harmful chemicals[8].

For agency nurses, we also ask:
How long have you worked for this agency? Which other agencies have you worked for and when?

This question provides some information about the stability of the nurse's work history. Unfortunately, some bad nurses agency-hop. When they are fired by one agency, they move on to another, with no real record of their performance following them. Knowing how many agencies a nurse has worked for might provide a clue as to whether you're dealing with a hopper. On the other hand, some agencies are not great to work for, and good nurses sometimes move around because they don't want to work for bad agencies.

What questions do you have for us?

This is the nurse's opportunity to interview you and determine whether your home is the best place for her or him. The questions the nurse asks should demonstrate that the nurse was listening to the information you provided during the interview and interest in your child's health.

The wrap-up

This is your chance to give a summary of what you are looking for in a nurse and what you are not looking for. Discuss what the next steps in the process will be, whether it's calling the agency or case manager or checking references. If you want to leave it open ended, you can tell the nurse that you are interviewing several candidates and you will make a decision soon. Good CEOs set clear expectations of what will happen next.

For a quick reference list of these interview questions, see the **Resources** section at the end of this book.

Evaluating the interview

Secondary to learning about a nurse's skills and experience, the interview gives you the chance to learn about the nurse's ability to communicate effectively, which is important since the nurse will need to interact with you, your child, and perhaps other nurses working in the home.

Red Flags

Be sure to watch for nonverbal communication and signs that you might not be getting the truth. Stammering, in the absence of a speech impediment, can signify dishonesty, as can general shiftiness. If a nurse seems uncomfortable, beyond the regular nerves people experience during a job interview, you might need to be concerned. Most of us know when people are trying to deceive us, so keep your eyes open for the signs. A nurse who is not forthcoming in the interview might turn into one of those horror stories we hear about.

Look for confidence when a nurse speaks about her or his experience. Usually, a nurse who has done a procedure hundreds of times talks about it differently than a newbie does. If experience is important to you, listen for signs that the nurse knows what she or he is doing.

The nurse should also be able to answer your questions without providing identifiers that violate HIPAA[6]. For example, they should not tell you the names, addresses, family details, specific identifying information, etc. of children for whom they have provided care. Not only is it illegal for a nurse to disclose this information to you, a nurse who tells you about personal details of other cases is likely to be just as loose with your child's private information.

Also, nurses wash their hands a lot. They understand that hand washing is the first line of defense against the spread of disease. Conscientious nurses will not touch your child without washing their hands first, even during an interview.

Check the paper trail

In addition to the interview, it's always a good idea to do a simple online search of the nurse you interviewed. Type their names into a search engine and see what comes up, paying special attention to social media accounts and anything that indicates criminal activity. Independent web services like 5starnurse.com can provide ratings for nurses based on the personal experiences of families.

You can always ask for references. If a nurse provides references, check them. You may even want to ask other nurses about the nurse you want to hire. The pediatric nursing community can be rather tightly knit, so it can be easy to find an informal reference.

Always check the status of the nurse's license, even if you are using an agency. Don't just depend on agencies to have the latest information about the nurses they hire. A simple check of the nurse's license status on your state's Board of Nursing website can alert you of major issues like a suspension or a revoked license.

Your decision about whether a nurse is a good fit for your child should be made with consideration of all that you know about the nurse. If you feel hesitant or concerned about any aspect of the

29

nurse's background, it's okay to keep searching. It's okay to be picky when you are selecting a nurse for your child. When you find a great nurse that will work well with your child, it will be well worth the wait.

CHAPTER 5

Communicating with your child's nurses

Now that you have the right people in place, your job as Home Care CEO is to communicate the mission and goals to the nurses and provide details on how to achieve them.

First things first: Contact information

I ask that each nurse give me her or his cell phone number, and I provide the nurse with our numbers. While some agencies object to families having direct contact with the nurse, my personal expectation is that if I leave my child with someone, I need to be able to contact that person at all times, and vice versa.

Communication book

A communication book can be an excellent tool for ensuring that all nurses know what is going on with your child. You can have nurses use the notebook daily or only when big changes occur. You can also have nurses use the book to request time off and to find other nurses to cover the missed shifts.

You might use a three-ring binder that has tabs for contact information (for your family members and the other nurses), medication changes, current goals, therapy activities, House Rules, daily schedules for your child, information about your child's medical supplies and equipment, and even reference material about your child's medical condition. Set the expectation that the notebook should be reviewed by nurses at the start of each shift.

> *We use a bound journal and date each entry in the book. In addition to the sections listed above, we have things like our Wi-Fi password, doctors' contact information and DME company phone number in the communication notebook. The book also serves as a great record of changes in our son's medical care, since the nurses and I make notes about his progress.*

You can also keep it simple with just a notebook and the sections that are most important for you and your child. For a guide on how to organize your communication book, see the **Resources** section at the end of this book.

Establishing House Rules

- Is it okay for your child's nurses to talk on their cell phones throughout their work shifts? How much is too much?
- Is texting or playing games on a device or laptop okay with you? What about reading, listening to music or singing?
- Can the nurse go outside to smoke during the shift?
- Do you expect the nurse to do light housework like dusting, dishes, sweeping, laundry or cleaning up toys?
- Can the nurse use the refrigerator and microwave?
- How do you expect the nurse to interact with the other members of the household or with family pets? Where does the nurse's authority begin and end when it comes to other children in the household?
- Do you want the nurse's advice on discipline or family issues?
- What can night nurses do to stay awake in your home?
- Where can nurses go or not go inside your home?

- Do you have concerns about nurses wearing shoes in the house?
- Do nurses bring their own tools and supplies (stethoscope, masks, gloves), or do you prefer that they use the ones in your home.
- How do nurses request time off, and how far in advance? Are they responsible for getting another nurse to cover the missed shift?

You will need to make decisions on House Rules like these and be consistent in enforcing the rules you set. You might have different rules, depending on the shift the nurse works. The rules you set should be based on the needs of your child and your family. If you don't want nurses talking loudly on the phone while you sleep, create a rule. If you want nurses to be within a certain distance of your child at all times, say so. Most importantly, put the rules in writing and make sure nurses know where to find them. You might use a communication book and tab a page for House Rules. Leave some space to add rules as you have new experiences. While you might think you don't have to say specifically that you don't want to hear a nurse's loud operatic singing at 4 a.m., it might happen, thus requiring you to add a new House Rule.

We allow our night nurses to play games and to text on their phones or tablets because our son is asleep for most of the night shift. However, he is awake, alert and ready to interact during the day shift, so we ask that nurses engage with him rather than with their technology, except in cases of emergency. We expect night nurses to keep the volume low on their devices or the TV so that our son can rest without distractions, while

33

during the day shift, the television is used for his educational videos. His care is always the first priority.

We ask that nurses use the stethoscope and supplies that we have in our home, rather than bringing their own supplies that may also be used in other homes, in order to minimize the risk of spreading illness.

Our son's nurses help with light housekeeping like cleaning equipment, washing dishes and syringes used during their shifts, vacuuming our son's room, and putting away his laundry.

When behavioral or disciplinary issues arise, our son's nurses redirect him to other activities, but they do not discipline in any way; they tell us about the behavior, and we develop a plan for how we and the nurses will address it in the future.

One of our most important House Rules is that everyone washes their hands before touching our son or anything in his room. Even if they showered at home, they wash up when they arrive at our house. I believe this rule alone has contributed tremendously to our son's health.

The partnership between nurses and families is based on mutual trust, and defining the boundaries and rules clearly will help everyone involved, especially your child.

Agency Rules

Agencies often have their own sets of rules for their nurses. Be aware of the agency's rules. Some will not allow nurses to use laptops at work, while others require that the nurse wear shoes at all times. If these rules conflict with your House Rules, you may have to be creative.

One of the agencies we use requires nurses to wear shoes at all times, but in our home, we remove outside shoes at the door and don't wear them throughout the house. To work around this rule, I have asked that nurses carry with them a pair of shoes that has not been worn outside. They change into these shoes when they enter our home. We also have shoe covers available for other people who need to enter our home, like therapists, equipment repair people and case managers.

Setting expectations

As the Home Care CEO, you will need to explain to your child's nurses what needs to be done and how you want it done. If there is a particular way that you handle your child's care, take time to explain and demonstrate that to the nurses, and be sure they take notes. Provide a lot of detail for how things are done, how long, how equipment should be cleaned and where items should be placed or put away.

For a while, we had an elaborate way of doing trach care for our son to prevent skin breakdown under his trach ties. We used a thin layer of ointment, followed by a light coating of cornstarch-based baby powder, before applying a six-inch by one-inch strip of Telfa (surgical wound dressing) under the trach tie. Once we discovered that this method kept our son's skin healthy, we taught each nurse how to do it and made notes about it in our communication book. Together, we were able to keep his skin healthy.

Setting clear expectations up front will save you headaches later because every nurse will know what you want. If you're ambitious, or just a neat freak, you may even want to type these expectations for each nurse or place them on a chart on the wall or in a communication book.

Over time, you might decide to change the way some things are done. When you make changes, notify every nurse of the new expectations so that you are all on the same page. Write down new instructions and be sure that all nurses have them. Communicating like a CEO requires planning and organization to get the results you want, and nurses learn to trust and value the communication.

In our home, we give nurses a detailed, hour-by-hour schedule chart that describes what takes place during the day and how we want each task done.

For a free download of a customizable hour-by-hour schedule chart, see the **Resources** section at the end of this book.

End-of-shift report

The information you request at the end of a nurse's shift will help you to determine what your child's current medical status and needs are. This list will differ based on your child's individual needs.

This is the list of end-of-shift report items that we use for our child who has a tracheostomy, a g-tube and mobility issues.

- When did he sleep and for how long? What was the quality of his sleep?
- What were his heart rate and oxygen saturation (sats) throughout the shift?
- What was his body temperature throughout the shift?
- What were his trach secretions like: amount (heavy/light), texture (foamy/frothy/creamy), color (yellow/white/blood-tinged/other)?

- What were his breath sounds like throughout the shift?
- When was he last changed (diaper/briefs or clothes)? How many wet or soiled diapers/briefs did he have during the shift?
- When did he last use the restroom? How many bowel movements did he have?
- When was he last repositioned?
- What activities did he do throughout the shift and for how long?
- Do you have any other concerns?
- When did he eat (if meal times are not predetermined)?

The answers to these questions allow a smooth transition of care from the nurse to the family caregiver or to the next nurse taking over. They provide a baseline for our son's condition and let us know if there are any immediate concerns that need to be addressed.

Enforcing HIPAA

Do you mind if your child's in-home nurse discusses your child's condition with other nurses or families? While HIPAA forbids this, you may find that some nurses are a lot more casual than others are with private information. If you value privacy, say so directly, and let each nurse know that you expect him or her to comply very strictly with the laws regarding the privacy of your child's information.

Managing quality

House Rules and schedules describe what should and should not be done, but managing quality is looking at *how* things are done and *how well* things are done for your child's care. Once again, setting expectations is absolutely necessary for you and for the nurses. Most nurses want to do well, so telling them what you expect is a way for them to measure their own progress. It also saves you time and effort; you reduce the likelihood that you will need to repeat your expectations over and over again if you have provided them up front. As the Home Care CEO, you are ultimately responsible for ensuring that each nurse meets your expectations for care, so it is your job to communicate those expectations.

- How long and where does your child sit, stand, play, nap and do therapy activities?
- What is your child's daily schedule, and how strict is it from day to day?
- How frequently does your child have diaper changes, suctioning, repositioning, temperature checks, etc.?
- Does your child take any controlled substances? What are your procedures for counting the medications after each shift and ensuring that they are accounted for?
- Should nurses notify you when supplies or medications are running low? Are they responsible for reordering the items?
- What maintenance or cleaning is required for your child's equipment? Do nurses do the cleaning?
- How frequently are wound dressings and medical devices (like colostomy pouches and wafers, tracheostomy tubes and feeding tubes) replaced or cleaned? Who does it?
- Does your child have recommended activities for various therapies? Will the nurse participate in these therapeutic activities?

All these questions relate to the quality of care your child receives, how closely that quality is managed, and by whom. You will need to communicate these expectations to each nurse so that everyone is on board with the mission of excellent care for your child.

Performance problems
Below is a list of common issues parents have with in-home nurses:
- Sleeping on the job
- Smoking during a shift (see MUI section)
- Overstepping boundaries, including intruding in family affairs or overriding parents' decisions on matters not related to safety
- Attendance and tardiness issues
- Personality conflicts
- Not following the House Rules or guidelines
- Neglect and/or abuse (see MUI section)
- Stealing (see MUI section)
- Not providing the appropriate level of care (see MUI section)

MUI – Major Unusual Incident
An MUI (major unusual incident) is an "alleged, suspected or actual occurrence of an incident when there is reason to believe the health and safety of an individual may be adversely affected and the individual may be placed at a reasonable risk of harm" [9].

MUIs include physical, sexual and verbal abuse or exploitation, injuries that prevent normal activities for more than two consecutive days (burns, cuts, broken bones, etc.), medical emergencies, incidents that require law enforcement intervention, and the failure to report any of these types of incidents[9]. Check your state's definition of MUI to be aware of all types of incidents that fall under this heading.

All case managers, nursing agencies, and social workers who work with your child should be notified of an MUI. Some MUIs may require the involvement of law enforcement. Many times, MUIs result in the termination of a nurse's employment.

If you suspect that a nurse is mistreating your child, stop allowing that nurse to care for your child immediately, and contact the appropriate authorities. Do not place your child's health or safety at risk by knowingly allowing an abusive or neglectful person to care for him or her.

Nipping it in the bud

Dealing with nurses can be frustrating at times, and it's normal to want to scream when a nurse calls in sick at the last minute or provides sloppy care for your child. In order to keep nurses aligned with your expectations for excellent care, communicating early and often about problems is the best way to keep problems from getting worse. Sitting a nurse down to talk about performance issues can be uncomfortable, especially for those of us who are non-confrontational. This is when you have to harness your inner CEO and remember that the mission of excellent care is more important than the emotions surrounding these conversations.

My sister, whose disability required her to have in-home nursing, once said about nurses, "If they start off bad, they'll only get worse." I have found this advice to be very true. Early on, I had difficulty voicing my needs or dissatisfaction with nurses. What I have learned along the way is that it's not about me or my discomfort. It's about the mission: ensuring the best possible care for my child. If a nurse is jeopardizing that mission, it is my goal to bring her or him back into alignment with it. I make notes about what I would like to see the nurse

40

do differently, talk through the notes with the nurse, and make sure the nurse understands what our needs are. Sometimes I type these notes and give a copy of the notes to the nurse.

How many strikes?

Whether or not you choose to let a nurse go depends on how the nurse's behavior affects your child and family, and whether or not you are willing to tolerate the behavior for the long term. However, any time an MUI occurs, you should seriously consider letting the nurse go.

Remember, the purpose of in-home nursing is to give parents a break and ease the stress of providing care for the child. If a nurse creates more work for you or makes you more stressed out, that nurse is not fulfilling the purpose of the job.

Choosing the right words

Choosing the right time and the right words to say when terminating a nurse's employment depends on the nature of the problem with the nurse and whether the nurse is an independent provider or agency nurse.

Letting agency nurses go

For agency nurses, the procedure is simple. Contact the agency's case manager and ask that the nurse not return to your home. You may want the agency to find a nurse to replace the one you want to get rid of, while you keep the nurse in the home until they find a replacement. If an MUI has occurred, however, the nurse will probably be removed from working in your home immediately.

Letting independent nurses go

In order to get rid of an independent nurse, you need to get your hands a little dirty. Some cases, like abuse, neglect or the inability to provide adequate care, may require you to ask a nurse to leave immediately or to call the authorities. Depending on the circumstances, you might be angry or upset with the nurse, but try to remain calm; maintain a physical distance from the nurse if you can. You can ask the nurse to leave by saying:

> *"We won't need you to finish your shift today. I will sign you out so you can go now, and we will not need you to come back."*

If at all possible, we try not to fire nurses while they are in our home. For safety reasons, and because it is hard to predict how people will react to being let go, we prefer to do it by phone. Our script for terminating a nurse's employment by phone is:

> *"We have decided to make some changes to ___'s nursing care, and we will not need you to return."*

If asked, you may choose to provide detailed reasons for your choice to let the nurse go.

By remaining calm and matter-of-fact, you can keep an emotional situation under control as you end a bad relationship.

Agency problems

Performance problems can apply not just to individual nurses, but also to agencies. Poor management of nurses, hard-to-reach agency staff, and bad scheduling practices are the most common problems parents have with agencies. Unfortunately, these problems plague small and large agencies. Even if there are very few nursing agencies to choose from in your area, this should not stop you from expecting quality service.

Know the contact people for the nursing agency, and have their numbers handy at all times. The director of nursing is usually the person to talk to when all others have failed. If an agency continues to create stress for you, talk to your child's Medicaid case manager about the agency. The case manager may be able to communicate on your behalf and get results for you. Since most agencies don't want to be seen in a bad light by case managers who work for the state's Medicaid administrators or Developmental Disabilities boards, you might notice a quick change if your child's case manager calls on your behalf.

When possible, you may choose to work with more than one agency or to employ independent nurses to ensure that all shifts are covered to your satisfaction.

Trusting your gut

Entrusting your child to someone else is huge, and when your child is medically fragile, this is even harder to do. Sometimes a little voice tells you it's just not right. Sometimes you don't even know why. At times, personalities don't mesh and a nurse just isn't right for your home. Other times, red flags let you know that a nurse doesn't have what it takes to meet your child's needs. Whatever the reason, trust your instincts. Trusting your gut works in both directions. Sometimes you just know a nurse is the right fit.

I have personally experienced both sides of listening to my instincts in terms of hiring or keeping nurses.

On one occasion, I interviewed a nurse who had lots of experience. During the initial visit in my home, she tried to touch my son without washing her hands, which was a red flag for me. Something about her didn't feel right to me, but I dismissed my doubts since she had the right experience. After working only two nights in our home, she committed a MUI, which we were fortunate to have on video. Needless to say, she did not return. I'm glad we caught it early, but I wish I had trusted that feeling that said, "Not this one."

A more positive example is when a very skilled agency nurse filled in one night soon after our son was discharged from the hospital. She was warm, caring and compassionate, and I was able to detect that in the one night she worked with our son. A few weeks later, I asked the agency about her, and she has been one of our son's nurses ever since.

Think of instinct as an unscientific, unquantifiable tool that can be used along with more concrete evaluations to make a well-rounded decision.

Keep Trying.

Don't be discouraged when it doesn't work out with the nurse you hire; just keep searching. CEOs don't have a meltdown when their newest employee doesn't hit the mark; they just try again until they find the right fit.

Our attitude when we find a new nurse is always, "we'll see how this goes." It may sound a little jaded, but it's actually a sign that we are open to whatever comes, good or bad. We don't place too much stock in any particular nurse being a perfect fit, so we just wait to see how the nurse works out. We know we can always make a different decision later.

44

CHAPTER 6

Remaining informed

Most people underestimate how much leadership and learning are connected. Staying up-to-date on treatments, equipment, research and current events can help you to identify ways to provide better care for your child [10].

No CEO operates in a bubble. They need to know what's going on in the world outside in order to plan for the future. In the same way, you will need to be aware of many moving parts that affect your child's care. When your child has a medical condition, you learn a new language of medical terms, and you learn so much about providing care. By continuing the learning process, you can work toward always receiving the best care for your child.

Parents of medically fragile children find themselves becoming experts in lots of different areas, including laws and regulations, research and treatments, and the specialties that support the health of their children. Some of the changes in these areas will inevitably affect in-home nursing care, so it is important to stay in the know.

As you seek new information for the care of your child, be careful to consider the source, especially online. Use reputable websites by the National Institutes of Health (NIH), Mayo Clinic and other research organizations that provide expert opinions. While blog sites and online support groups are useful, be mindful that each child is unique. When you find innovative treatments or new information, talk to your child's physicians, specialists and nurses about them before taking action.

When we connect to others and work together, we find that the world looks a bit brighter and things don't seem as complicated. Join online groups, local support groups, hospital family advisory councils, and condition-specific groups (such as Muscular Dystrophy Association or Down Syndrome Association) that can keep you connected and aware, to the extent that your time allows.

Keep in mind that involvement in these organizations is intended to energize and empower you to manage your child's care. Too much involvement can burn you out, so choose carefully based upon an organization's relevance for your child and its effectiveness at meeting your needs. Don't go overboard; you still need to balance time and attention for yourself and your family.

Learn from your child's nurses

While your goal is to learn as much as you can, you can tire yourself out trying to learn everything. This is where your child's nurse can be a great partner. Having in-home nursing requires mutual respect: you respect the expertise of the nurses, and they respect your child and the way you want things done for your child in your home. Your child's nurses come with knowledge and experience, and you can learn a lot from them. They have often provided care for children with complex medical needs for years or decades, making them a great resource. The wealth of knowledge they bring can help you provide better care for your child.

At the same time, each child is different, and nurses should honor your child's individuality, along with your wishes for how you want to manage your child's care. There is not one single right way to do things, so you learn to do what works for your child. Nurses are there to support you, care for your child and provide expertise and information to keep your child healthy.

CHAPTER 7

The big picture

CEOs have to adapt, and the world of in-home nursing involves perpetual change.

When our son was preparing to be discharged from the hospital with home nursing, we were told that it could take up to a year to establish a stable in-home nursing staff. We were astounded and thought that seemed like ages, and we were confident that it wouldn't take us that long. It took us 11 ½ months to get a stable staff of nurses who met our son's needs to our satisfaction. Shortly after the one-year mark, one nurse needed to reduce her hours, sending our lovely sense of stability right out the window.

It is important to have realistic expectations of in-home nursing. In-home nursing is usually not a cure-all that will solve all complications related to the care of your medically fragile child. Even with in-home nursing, you may see differences in the workloads of people in your household; moms tend to take on more of the caregiving role. Caregivers may have to reduce work hours, change shifts, or change jobs. Sometimes, your child's nursing staff will be stable and predictable, which may be followed by periods of flux. This is normal. In fact, if your child comes home with a stable staff of nurses that remains stable for years without interruption, you might be a family of unicorns.

When you are dealing with human beings, you inevitably have

to deal with the uncertainties and complications of their lives, some of which will affect you and your family. When a nurse is sick or a nurse's child becomes ill, or when a nurse has to move or take on additional patients, it will affect your household. As a Home Care CEO, you will need to respond to changes in a way that keeps your mission at the center of everything.

Managing setbacks

Every CEO has moments that don't feel like success. There will definitely be times when you don't feel like you're in control of the home nursing situation, and that is natural. Managing in-home nursing is not always easy. It can be terribly frustrating sometimes, and it can take a while to feel like everything is under control, but success is possible.

Take a deep breath, and focus on the mission. Every decision should be guided by what is best for your child and family.

Signs of success

As in any company, the CEO is ultimately held responsible for failure and success. You guide the decisions because you are managing the care of *your* child in *your* home.

Your success as a Home Care CEO is judged by your Board of Directors and stockholders, your child and your family. If your child's health is stable or improving, if your family feels less stressed, if you are caring for yourself and your family in a way that is somewhat balanced most of the time, if you are all enjoying life in spite of the challenges, you can count that as success. Your bonus is work-life satisfaction that allows you to feel recharged and fulfilled. As the Home Care CEO, you have the power to achieve the mission of excellent care for your child.

REFERENCES

1 McMahon, Colin. "Pediatric Long term Care." Grand Rounds, Sept, 2009. Women and Children's Hospital of Buffalo.

2 Hogan, Dennis P. *Family Consequences of Children's Disabilities*. New York: Russell Sage Foundation, 2012. Google Book Search. Web. 16 Jan 2015.

3 Sobsey, Dick. "Marital stability and marital satisfaction in families of children with disabilities: Chicken or egg?" *Developmental Disabilities Bulletin 32.1* (2004): 62-83. Print.

4 "Medicaid Benefits." *Medicaid.gov*. Centers for Medicare & Medicaid Services. n.d. Web. 27 Jan 2015.

5 "Glossary." *LongTermCare.gov*. U.S. Department of Health and Human Services. n.d. Web. 27 January 2015.

6 "Health Information Privacy." *HHS.gov*. U.S. Department of Health and Human Services. n.d. Web. 27 January 2015.

7 "Health Effects of Secondhand Smoke." *Smoking and Tobacco Use*. Centers for Disease Control and Prevention. n.d Web. 27 Jan 2015.

8 Burton, Adrian. "Does the Smoke Ever Really Clear? Thirdhand Smoke Exposure Raises New Concerns." Environmental Health Perspectives 119(2): A70-A74. Web. 27 Jan 2015.

9 "Major Unusual Incidents: Understanding the MUI Reporting System." Ohio Department of Developmental Disabilities. n.d. 27 January 2015.

10 Reid, J.C., Kardash, C.A.M., Robinson, R.D., and Scholes, R.J. "Comprehension in patient literature: The importance of text and reader characteristics." *Health Communication 6(4):* 327-335. Print.

RESOURCES

Organizing your communication book

A binder that allows you to add and remove pages easily is a good place to start for your communication book.

Materials you will need
- A three-ringed binder or a blank notebook or journal
- Blank tabs that you can label
- Your child's basic medical information, surgery dates, health goals
- Contact information for people involved in your child's care
- Information about your child's medical equipment

Contact information
- Phone numbers and email addresses for family members involved in your child's care. Include your home address so that nurses can provide it to emergency responders if necessary.
- Contact information for all nurses who work with your child
- Contact information for physicians
- Contact information for therapists

Introduction
Include your child's date of birth, major health concerns, medical devices or equipment, limitations, and personality traits.

Current goals
This section will need to be updated periodically, based on your child's growth and development. Try to update it every 3-6 months. Keeping a word processing document that you can change quickly and print is a simple option.

Daily schedule
In addition to keeping a chart on the wall, you may decide to include a daily schedule in the communication book, detailing

which activities, treatments, medications or therapies are completed and at what time.

Medication changes

When medications are ordered or changed, include a copy of the prescription in this section. You may also make multiple copies so the nurses can keep copies.

Therapy activities

If therapists have suggested a range of therapeutic activities for your child, list them here or print out activities from the internet or Pinterest that you would like the nurses to do with your child. This will give them guidance on how to spend their time with your child and support his or her needs.

House Rules

Your rules and expectations for your home and your child's nurses should be outlined here. Leave space to add more rules. This is another section that you might choose to type and print, making changes as needed.

Information about your child's medical supplies and equipment

If you have hard copies of equipment manuals for your child's equipment, you can keep them in your communication book. In our home, we download these manuals to our son's tablet so nurses can access them when a problem arises. You might also list the name and phone number of your durable medical equipment (DME) provider so nurses can contact the company if there are equipment or supply problems.

Reference material about your child's medical condition

If your child has a rare condition, you might find that nurses have not encountered it before. You may wish to provide some information from the National Institutes of Health (NIH), which has a list of medical conditions on its website.

Interview questions for in-home nurses

1. Tell me about yourself.

2. Tell me about your experience caring for a child with _____.

3. Tell me about your pediatric experience.

4. What do you like most and least about home nursing?

5. Why did you leave your last case? Have you ever been fired or asked to leave a case?

6. Thinking about the families you have worked with in the past, what would they say about your attendance and timeliness?

7. Can you tell me about a time when you dealt with an emergency with a patient? What happened, what did you do, and what was the outcome?

8. What is your availability to work? Are you willing to fill in for other nurses if necessary? Are there days or times when you are absolutely not available?

9. Besides carrying out the doctor's orders in the care plan, how else do you assist or support the children and families on the cases you work?

10. Tell me about a situation where you disagreed with a parent about the appropriate way to care for their child. How did you handle it?

11. Do you smoke?

12. How long have you worked for this agency? Which other agencies have you worked for and when?

13. What questions do you have for us?

Hour-by-hour wall chart

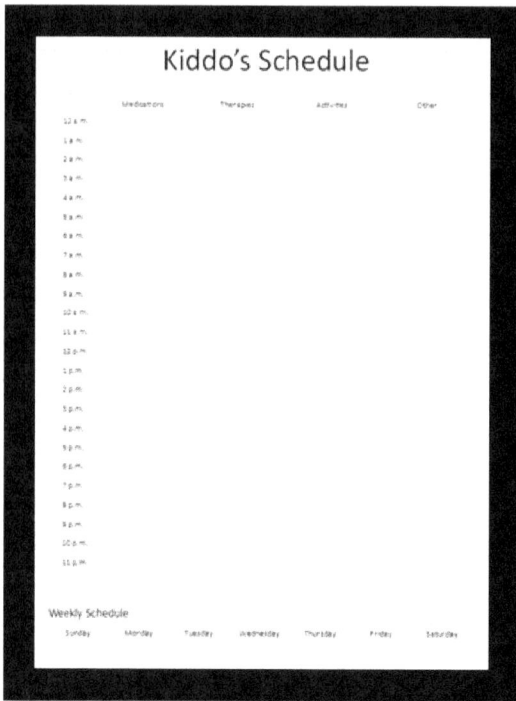

Download your free, customizable chart here:
http://bit.ly/1bBrwgU

You can change the headings, add a background photo and personalize it with your child's name.

You might choose to type in your child's schedule and print it on regular paper for the communication book, or you can go bigger. We saved our blank chart as a PDF file and had it printed on 28"x36" laminated paper so we could use it as a dry erase poster and update it easily.

www.ingramcontent.com/pod-product-compliance
Lightning Source LLC
LaVergne TN
LVHW051429080426
835508LV00022B/3315